CASTOR OIL FOR BEGINNERS

The Comprehensive Wisdom and Wellness Guide For Good Healthy Living

Heather J. Neilson

TABLE OF CONTENT

INTRODUCTION

A woman named Lily lived in a busy metropolis,surrounded by technology and a fast-paced rhythm of existence.

She was a modern-day go-getter who negotiated the business world with tenacity and elegance. Yet, underneath her confident demeanor, Lily endured a series of health issues that appeared to throw a pall over her colorful personality.

Irregular menstrual periods were a frequent companion, disrupting her daily routine. Lily frequently found herself fighting with her body's unpredictable nature, a battle that stretched beyond her personal life and into her professional obligations.

The illusive equilibrium she sought appeared to slide through her fingers like sand.

Her problems were exacerbated by her hair, which had previously been glossy but was now subdued by low quality and a discouraging proclivity for breaking. Lily's appearance in the mirror reflected her mental struggle, as seen by the blotches on her face and skin.

The ongoing fight with imperfections made her feel self-conscious and yearn for the dazzling skin she used to take for granted.

Lily's pain was exacerbated by problems with ingestion and constipation. The daily grind had taken its toll on her digestive system, leaving her lethargic and bloated. Joint aches were an unwanted companion, a reminder of hours spent sitting in the same position, working away at her computer in search of professional achievement.

Amid this maze of health issues, Lily discovered an unexpected savior: castor oil. Castor oil, hailed as a miracle for its numerous advantages, became a beacon of hope in Lily's quest to rediscover her best self. Initially skeptical, she adapted this old cure to her modern lifestyle.

As the weeks went by, Lily observed a transformational difference. Her monthly periods were regular, restoring a sense of order in her life.

Her hair's formerly weak strands began to reclaim their former splendor, each follicle endowed with unexpected vitality. The blemishes on her face gradually vanished, revealing a glowing complexion that represented both exterior attractiveness and interior energy.

Castor oil's influence went beyond surface-level changes. Lily received relief from ingesting and constipation difficulties, demonstrating the oil's holistic therapeutic capabilities. Her joint troubles faded into memory, allowing her to reclaim her mobility and vibrancy.

Lily's transformation from a lady struggling with health issues to the personification of her best self demonstrated the power of an age-old treatment in a modern environment.

Castor oil, once banished to the shadows of old knowledge, has resurfaced as a modern elixir, restoring Lily to the bright, confident woman she was destined to be.

Chapter 1: Unveiling Castor Oil's Ancient Wisdom

Castor oil, a time-honored elixir known for its astonishing flexibility, dates back to ancient civilizations. Exploring the profound knowledge contained in its application reveals a rich tapestry of historical relevance and therapeutic advantages.

Castor oil has been used in medicine since ancient Egypt and is known for its powerful therapeutic powers. Cleopatra supposedly used it as a beauty routine, demonstrating its usefulness beyond traditional medicines.

Across cultures, from India to China, this oil was revered for its cleansing and detoxifying properties.The ancient Greeks recognized the potential of castor oil and used it for a variety of purposes.

Renowned physicians like Hippocrates praised its potential to improve intestinal health and treat skin issues.

The knowledge of castor oil extended to ancient Ayurvedic treatments, where it was revered for its ability to promote total wellbeing.

Castor oil remained a staple of apothecary and herbalist treatments throughout medieval Europe. Its medicinal effects extended beyond direct use, and it became a mainstay in tonics and liniments.

Castor oil was portrayed as a sign of energy and well-being in the annals of time due to the holistic approach to health that persisted throughout history.

Fast forward to the present day, and the traditional knowledge of castor oil persists. As contemporary science explores further into its composition, we uncover an abundance of vital fatty acids and antioxidants that contribute to its rejuvenating powers.

From beauty regimens to holistic health practices, castor oil smoothly integrates into our lives, retaining the essence of old traditions in an ever-changing world.

Castor oil's voyage through time reveals not only its durability but also the eternal knowledge contained beneath its viscous depths.

Whether used as a beauty elixir, digestive aid, or holistic cure, castor oil exemplifies the continuing link between ancient knowledge and modern well-being.

Tracing Castor Oil's Timeless Roots

Castor oil is a versatile and long-lasting elixir with a rich history that is inextricably linked to human civilization.

Its origins may be traced back to ancient Egypt, when it was highly valued for its therapeutic virtues and used for a variety of cosmetic purposes. Castor oil's extraordinary journey spans time, weaving through many civilizations and leaving an unmistakable impression.

The ancient Egyptians prized castor oil not just for its purported therapeutic properties but also as a critical component in embalming procedures. Its viscosity and preservation properties make it an invaluable chemical for preserving the deceased.

As trade routes increased, castor oil crossed continents and made its way into

Ayurvedic medicine in India, where it was valued for its purgative effects and as a treatment for a variety of diseases.

The Mediterranean area, with its many civilizations, witnessed the incorporation of castor oil into traditional medicine. The Greeks and Romans knew its laxative properties and valued its usage in skincare treatments.

This versatile oil traveled down the Silk Road until it reached China, where it became an essential component of traditional Chinese medicine.

During the Middle Ages, castor oil's reputation as a strong treatment spread throughout Europe. It was popular among herbalists and healers, who recommended it for anything from stomach difficulties to skin concerns.

Its popularity lasted throughout the Renaissance and the Age of Exploration, when it became a common ingredient in apothecaries and medical gardens.

Castor oil's uses in the contemporary period have moved beyond traditional medicine. Because of its unusual chemical makeup, it has uses in a wide range of sectors, including cosmetics and manufacturing.

The robust roots of castor oil continue to flourish, responding to society's changing requirements, and its timeless attraction remains in the modern world.

Castor oil's long history demonstrates its lasting value. From ancient rites to current enterprises, its roots have dug deep into human history, creating an incredible legacy that is still unfolding.

The Intricate Chemistry Behind Castor Oil's Magic

Castor oil, an apparently simple material, has an intricate chemistry that reveals its mystical qualities. Castor oil is a triglyceride made mostly of ricinoleic acid.

This particular fatty acid accounts for approximately 90% of the oil's composition and is responsible for its amazing properties. Ricinoleic acid is not a common component in most vegetable oils; hence, castor oil stands out among natural medicines.

The magic starts with castor oil's ability to penetrate deeply into the skin. Ricinoleic acid facilitates this by increasing the oil's solubility in both water and oil, boosting absorption.

Castor oil, once ingested, increases the creation of prostaglandins, hormone-like molecules that play critical roles in a variety of physiological processes.

This stimulation enhances the oil's anti-inflammatory and analgesic qualities, making it a popular option for pain relief and inflammation reduction.

Castor oil has antibacterial qualities that attack germs and fungi. This makes it a significant tool for treating a variety of skin disorders, including acne and fungal infections.

Its capacity to hydrate and nourish the skin expands its usefulness, encouraging healthy skin in a variety of ways.

Beyond its outward usage, castor oil's complex chemistry extends to its internal use. When consumed, ricinoleic acid functions as a natural laxative by attaching to intestinal receptors and promoting bowel movements. This has resulted in castor oil's historical usage as a cure for constipation, although caution is advised owing to its strong effects.

The complex chemistry of ricinoleic acid is what gives castor oil its enchantment. Castor oil's versatility, ranging from skin penetration to anti-inflammatory, antibacterial, and laxative effects, has made it a traditional medicine mainstay.

Understanding the science behind this natural elixir helps us appreciate its many uses in boosting health and well-being.

Dispelling Myths and Embracing Realities oil

Castor oil has long been surrounded by myths and misconceptions, which frequently obscure its genuine advantages. Let us cut through the myths and embrace the truths of this versatile oil.

Myth 1: Castor oil is only for hair growth.
Reality: While castor oil is well-known for stimulating hair growth, its applications extend well beyond the domain of beauty.

It is an effective treatment for a variety of skin diseases due to its anti-inflammatory and antibacterial qualities. Castor oil is a flexible treatment that may be used to soothe inflamed skin or cure acne.

Myth 2: Castor oil is too thick for the skin.
Reality: While some may be concerned about castor oil's viscosity, it is precisely this

thickness that makes it a good emollient. When used in moderation, it seals in moisture and keeps the skin moisturized without blocking pores. The idea that it is overly heavy is a misconception; the trick is to use it wisely.

Myth 3: Castor Oil Isn't for the Face
Castor oil, contrary to common perception, may be extremely beneficial to the skin. It penetrates deep into the skin, increasing collagen formation and minimizing fine wrinkles.

It's an effective, natural way to counteract aging symptoms, making it an important part of your skincare regimen.

Myth 4: All castor oils are created. The quality of castor oil varies greatly. Choose cold-pressed, hexane-free variants to assure the purest quality of this oil. Unrefined castor oil has more nutrients and is free of toxic compounds, making it a healthier option.

Myth 5: Castor oil is harmful when consumed. Reality: Food-grade castor oil has been used for generations as a natural treatment for a variety of diseases. In moderation, it may be a healthy supplement to your diet. However, always speak with a healthcare expert before implementing it internally.

Dispelling these fallacies helps us to fully understand castor oil's actual potential. Accept the facts, investigate its various applications, and let this natural elixir become a mainstay in your wellness regimen.

Chapter 2: Selecting Your Castor Elixir

To achieve the best outcomes, selecting the proper castor oil, often known as castor elixir, requires careful consideration of a number of aspects.

First, choose cold-pressed castor oil, which contains more nutrients than heat-extracted oils. Cold-pressing maintains the oil's integrity and natural characteristics, making it an excellent choice for skincare and haircare.

Consider the color of the castor oil; high-quality castor oil is usually light yellow. This means that it is pure and poorly treated.

Avoid oils that are extremely black or hazy, since they may contain contaminants or additives. Additionally, check for organic and hexane-free solutions to guarantee that no toxic chemicals are included in the finished product.

Castor oil's viscosity is very important in hair treatments. Choose a medium-to-thick consistency for efficient application and absorption. Thicker oils are ideal for deep conditioning and restoring dry, damaged hair.

Check the product label for any extra components. Some castor oil formulations incorporate additions such as vitamin E or other natural oils, which increase the overall benefits.

If you have sensitive skin or special requirements, go for a pure, single-ingredient castor oil.Consider the packaging for the castor oil. Choose items packaged in dark glass bottles to keep the oil from light, which can impair its quality over time.

A bottle with a dropper or pump facilitates application and reduces waste.

Check user reviews and testimonials to determine the product's usefulness. Real-world experiences can shed light on the oil's effectiveness for a variety of applications, including encouraging hair growth, hydrating skin, and reducing joint pain.

Choose cold-pressed, pale yellow, organic, hexane-free castor oil with a medium to thick viscosity.

Check for other helpful components, use a dark glass container with a handy dispenser, and examine genuine user reviews to make an informed selection about your castor elixir.

Navigating a Sea of Varieties

Navigating the huge array of castor oil variations needs a keen eye and a thorough grasp of its many applications.

Castor oil is well-known for its flexibility, and it comes in a variety of forms, each customized to specific purposes. From pharmaceutical-grade to industrial applications, selecting the proper variation is critical for the best outcomes.

One important factor to examine is the quality of castor oil. Pharmaceutical-grade castor oil, extracted using precise methods, is perfect for medical and cosmetic applications.

It guarantees a high degree of purity, devoid of contaminants that might impair its efficiency. Industrial-grade variations, on the other hand, are valued for their durability in applications like lubricants and coatings.

Castor oil's functioning is highly dependent on its viscosity. Low-viscosity variations are used for applications requiring high fluidity, such as hydraulic fluids or paint bases.

In contrast, high-viscosity castor oil is useful in businesses that require thicker lubricants or as a key component in the creation of certain polymers.

Another important aspect is the degree of fineness. Cold-pressed castor oil keeps more of the seeds' natural components, making it appropriate for organic cosmetics.

In contrast, refined castor oil, obtained through extensive processing, is favored in applications that need a neutral, odorless, and colorless product.

Geographical origin adds to the diversity of castor oil. Varieties from various areas may have distinct traits that influence their usefulness for certain applications. Indian castor oil, for example, is known for its high ricinoleic acid concentration, making it a popular ingredient in several medicinal compositions.

Navigating the sea of castor oil types requires a thorough awareness of their purity, viscosity, refining degree, and geographical origin.

Tailoring the choice to the desired use guarantees that this adaptable oil may be used to its full capacity in a variety of sectors.

Quality Check: Ensuring Purity and Potency

Ensuring the quality of castor oil is critical for both customers and manufacturers. The potency and purity of castor oil are critical factors in determining its usefulness in a variety of applications. From cosmetics to industrial applications, strict quality criteria are required.

To ensure purity, the castor oil manufacturing process undergoes stringent quality tests. The absence of impurities and adequate extraction procedures are critical. Quality control begins at the cultivation stage, ensuring that the Ricinus communis plant is grown under ideal circumstances.

This involves monitoring soil quality, adopting organic agricultural techniques, and minimizing the use of hazardous chemicals.

Advanced extraction technologies are used to reduce contaminants. Cold pressing yields high-quality castor oil while keeping its natural qualities. Rigorous filtration methods further eradicate any leftover particles, resulting in a pure final product.

Potency is another important feature of castor oil quality.

The concentration of important beneficial chemicals, such as ricinoleic acid, impacts its efficacy. Advanced testing procedures are used to evaluate the oil's chemical composition and ensure that it satisfies the specified potency levels.

This guarantees its efficacy in conventional medical uses while also improving its performance in cosmetic and industrial compositions.

Third-party testing provides an additional degree of validation. Independent laboratories undertake thorough studies to validate purity and potency claims.

This honest approach earns consumers' trust by ensuring the quality of the castor oil they are using.

Castor oil quality must be maintained through a complete method that includes cultivation, extraction, and third-party certification.

Purity and potency are more than just buzzwords; they are the cornerstones of a dependable and successful product, making high-quality castor oil an invaluable tool in a variety of sectors.

Organic vs. Cold-Pressed Dilemma

Organic castor oil and cold-pressed castor oil create a quandary for consumers looking for the finest alternative for their skincare and haircare regimens.

Both methods of manufacturing have unique properties that might affect the quality and advantages of the oil.

Organic castor oil is produced without using synthetic pesticides, herbicides, or chemical fertilizers. This guarantees that the oil is free of hazardous residues and encourages more ecologically friendly growing practices.

The organic certification also ensures that the whole manufacturing chain follows stringent criteria.

Cold-pressed castor oil, on the other hand, is derived by pressing castor beans at low temperatures, usually less than 120°F (49°C). This procedure tries to retain the oil's natural qualities by avoiding high temperatures, which can destroy its nutritional value.

Cold-pressing is commonly used to preserve the oil's particular makeup, which includes important fatty acids and vitamins.

Individual interests and priorities determine whether to choose organic or cold-pressed castor oil. If environmental sustainability and the lack of synthetic chemicals are important considerations, organic castor oil is the better alternative.

It is consistent with a holistic approach to personal care and a dedication to promoting environmentally responsible methods.

Cold-pressed castor oil, on the other hand, may be preferred by individuals who want to preserve the inherent nutrients of the oil. The mild extraction technique preserves healthy components, perhaps improving hair and skin health.

In the case of castor oil, the choice between organic and cold-pressed comes down to personal beliefs and desired goals.

Whether one chooses the environmental sensitivity of organic farming or the nutritional preservation of cold-pressing, both methods address various facets of a thoughtful and health-conscious lifestyle.

Chapter 3: The Art of Healing with Castor Oil

Castor oil, a versatile and time-tested medicine, is a shining light in the field of natural healing. Its therapeutic benefits go beyond simple lubrication, diving into a comprehensive approach to well-being.

Castor oil, which harnesses the strong qualities of the Ricinus communis plant, emerges as an artistic healer.

First and foremost, castor oil is a skincare champion. It easily hydrates, rejuvenates, and calms the skin due to its high fatty acid content. Its emollient properties penetrate deeply, resulting in a soft and luminous complexion.

This makes it an artistic elixir that removes dryness, wrinkles, and imperfections, revealing a canvas of natural beauty.

Furthermore, castor oil is well-known for its hair-care benefits. Its moisturizing touch promotes hair development, strengthens follicles, and soothes a dry scalp.

 This golden elixir not only promotes lush trees but also treats dandruff and broken ends. The creativity is in its capacity to turn drab threads into a flood of life.

Castor oil is well-known for its ability to relieve pain and inflammation in addition to its cosmetic properties. Its anti-inflammatory effects make it a soothing salve for tight muscles and joints.

This natural therapy gently rubs away tension, giving a sensation of peace and calm. It's a painting of healing strokes made with the gentle touch of nature.

Castor oil's therapeutic properties extend to the digestive system. It is a moderate laxative that helps regulate bowel motions and promotes gut health. Its delicate yet efficient approach to digestion distinguishes it as a medicine founded on balance and harmony.

The multidimensional approach to well-being is what distinguishes castor oil-based treatments. Its therapeutic strokes produce a masterpiece of holistic health, including skincare, haircare, pain alleviation, and digestive harmony.

Accept the time-honored heritage of castor oil therapy and discover the canvas of wellbeing that nature has generously given us.

Skincare Miracles Unleashed

Unlock the key to glowing skin with Castor oil, a skincare marvel. Castor Oil, known for its many advantages, has emerged as a skincare powerhouse, providing a unique combination of nourishment and renewal.

First and foremost, Castor Oil is a natural moisturizer that extends beyond surface hydration. Its creamy texture penetrates deeply into the skin, trapping in moisture and leaving it supple and silky.
Say goodbye to dry, flaky skin as Castor Oil works its magic to restore your skin's natural moisture balance.

Castor oil also has strong anti-inflammatory qualities, making it an ideal choice for calming sensitive skin. Castor Oil soothes redness, irritation, and inflammation, resulting in a smoother and more pleasant skin.

One of Castor Oil's distinguishing properties is its ability to boost collagen formation. Collagen is the structural protein that keeps the skin elastic and firm.

Regular usage of Castor Oil can help reduce the appearance of fine lines and wrinkles, revealing a more young and vibrant complexion.

Castor Oil's antimicrobial characteristics might help you get rid of obstinate acne. It fights acne-causing germs, reducing outbreaks and creating a brighter complexion.

Furthermore, its low comedogenic rating guarantees that it hydrates without blocking pores, making it appropriate for a variety of skin types.

Castor oil isn't just for facial treatment; it's also a multipurpose elixir for hair and nails.

Massaging Castor Oil into your scalp stimulates hair development and strengthens strands, while putting it to your nails nourishes cuticles and promotes better nail growth.

Castor oil is more than simply a skincare cure; it is a complete answer for individuals looking for revolutionary outcomes.

Accept the skincare wonders unleashed by castor oil and bask in the beautiful, renewed beauty it provides for your skin.

Alleviating Aches through Castor Oil Packs

Castor oil packs have acquired popularity as a natural and efficient method of pain management.

Castor oil, extracted from the seeds of the Ricinus communis plant, is well-known for its anti-inflammatory and analgesic qualities. When administered in the form of packs, it can provide relief from a variety of symptoms.

Castor oil packs are made by soaking a piece of cloth in oil and applying it to the afflicted region. This simple yet effective therapy improves circulation, reduces inflammation, and relaxes tight muscles.

The heat created by the pack increases blood flow, which facilitates the passage of nutrients and oxygen to the damaged tissues, aiding healing.

One of the primary advantages of castor Oil packs is their adaptability in treating many forms of pain. Whether you have muscular tightness, joint pain, or menstrual cramps, the packs may be placed in the affected region for focused treatment.

As a result, castor oil packs are a popular choice for people looking for a natural and non-invasive way to treat pain.

Furthermore, castor oil has been associated with detoxifying properties. The packs are said to stimulate the lymphatic system, promoting the elimination of toxins from the body.

This cleansing action can improve general health and may be especially useful for people who suffer from chronic pain.

It's important to remember that, while castor oil packs provide a natural option for pain relief, they're not a one-size-fits-all answer. Individuals with specific medical ailments or concerns should contact a healthcare expert before introducing castor oil packs into their daily regimen.

Using castor oil's medicinal capabilities in packs offers a simple and innovative way to relieve discomfort.

The natural components in castor oil, along with the focused application of the packs, result in a comprehensive approach to pain treatment that many people find helpful and calming.

Ancient Wisdom in Modern Medicine

Ancient knowledge smoothly integrates with modern medicine, revealing time-tested cures that remain relevant in today's health practices. One of these riches is castor oil, which is extracted from the Ricinus communis plant.

Castor oil has been valued since antiquity for its varied medicinal effects. From Egypt to India, ancient healers used it to treat a wide range of diseases.

Fast forward to the current day, and scientific investigation has confirmed many of these historical statements.

One of castor oil's main characteristics is its anti-inflammatory properties. Modern medicine acknowledges its capacity to treat joint pain, arthritis, and muscular soreness.

The oil's ricinoleic acid concentration, a strong anti-inflammatory agent, is critical in lowering inflammation and delivering comfort in a way that is consistent with traditional healers' beliefs.

Furthermore, castor oil's antibacterial and antifungal qualities make it an effective opponent of skin problems.

Its topical use promotes wound healing and soothes skin irritations, confirming old wisdom that recognized the oil as a powerful remedy for skin ailments.

Castor oil has traditionally been used to treat constipation. The oil's laxative properties may be traced back to ancient therapeutic techniques, when it was used to encourage regular bowel movements.

This is consistent with current research on the oil's effects on the digestive system, providing a natural alternative for people seeking relief.

Castor oil serves as a witness to the long-lasting efficacy of traditional therapies as the fusion of ancient wisdom and contemporary medicine continues.

Its numerous advantages highlight the compatibility between age-old wisdom and cutting-edge medical knowledge, promoting a comprehensive approach to health that transcends time.

Chapter 4: Infusing Wellness into Daily Life

Integrating natural therapies such as castor oil into daily life allows for a more holistic approach to health. Castor oil, known for its numerous advantages, may be easily included in a daily regimen.

Its high fatty acid content supports skin and hair health by serving as a powerful moisturizer and nourishing agent.

Begin your wellness journey by adding castor oil to your skincare routine. Its antibacterial characteristics help fight acne and decrease inflammation, leaving your skin refreshed.

A nightly application can reduce fine lines and wrinkles, resulting in a more youthful appearance. Massage a tiny quantity over your face and watch the magic happen as you wake up with glowing skin.

Castor oil is your hair's greatest friend when it comes to gorgeous locks. Its moisturizing effects strengthen hair follicles, reducing breakage and promoting growth.

A monthly castor oil hair mask helps rejuvenate dull, damaged hair, making it smooth and manageable. Massaging this liquid gold into your scalp and strands will eliminate frizz and restore a natural shine.

Castor oil also does wonders for interior health. Including it in your diet improves digestion, relieves constipation, and promotes gut health.

A teaspoon of castor oil on an empty stomach might stimulate your digestive system and promote overall health.

Embrace castor oil's calming benefits for muscle and joint wellness. Its anti-inflammatory properties make it a great treatment for painful muscles and joint discomfort.

A gentle massage with heated castor oil promotes comfort and reduces stress, making it an excellent complement to your relaxation regimen.

Castor oil is an easy and effective way to include wellness into your everyday routine. This natural elixir improves your general well-being in a variety of ways, including skincare, haircare, digestion, and relaxation.

Accept the transformational properties of castor oil for a healthier, more vibrant living.

Radiance Rituals with Castor Oil

Radiance rituals allow you to experience castor oil's transformational effect in your beauty regimen.

Castor oil, derived from the seeds of the Ricinus communis plant, has emerged as a multipurpose elixir known for its outstanding health benefits.

Nourish your hair for a more vibrant look. Radiance Rituals incorporates castor oil into their products to profoundly nourish and moisturize your hair.

This natural emollient smoothes the hair cuticle, resulting in a glossy sheen that exudes vitality. Say goodbye to split ends and hello to a vivid, rejuvenated mane.

Radiance Rituals offers castor oil-infused elixirs for enhancing brows and eyelashes. The oil's rich nutrients help to strengthen and thicken lashes and brows, resulting in a stunning frame that naturally draws attention.

Castor Oil has skin-rejuvenating effects that can reveal glowing skin. Radiance Rituals combines this natural marvel into their skincare products, which promote moisture and solve common skin issues.

Embrace a healthy-looking complexion free of dryness and irritation.

Radiance Rituals' cleaning products use the purifying properties of castor oil.

 Experience a mild yet powerful cleansing that eliminates pollutants and makeup without depriving your skin of its natural moisture. Enjoy a fresh complexion that sets the tone for your bright attractiveness.

Enhance your Radiance Rituals experience by caring for your nails and cuticles. Castor oil's emollient qualities help to promote strong, healthy nails while also softening cuticles. Create manicure-worthy hands that demonstrate your dedication to total well-being.

Incorporate radiant rituals into your everyday routine to improve your self-care experience. With castor oil as its foundation, this collection reveals the secrets of glowing hair, attractive eyes, bright skin, and flawless nails.

With Radiance Rituals, you may experience the beauty of simplicity while allowing your natural radiance to come through.

Navigating Internal Use Safely

To guarantee safety and maximize benefits, it is necessary to take a deliberate approach while using castor Oil internally.

Castor oil, which is well-known for its therapeutic characteristics, must be used with caution to maximize its benefits without jeopardizing one's health. Here's a guide to a safe interior adventure.

1. Quality Matters:
Choose high-quality, cold-pressed castor oil devoid of additives and contaminants. Choosing organic alternatives assures purity and reduces the chance of contamination.

2. Dosage precision is crucial when taking castor oil internally. Begin with a little amount and progressively increase while monitoring your body's reaction. Consistency is essential for measuring

performance without overwhelming your system.

3. ***Purposeful Consumption:*** Identify internal advantages such as digestive health, immunological support, and more. Tailor the dosage and frequency to your personal health objectives.

4. ***Mixing Techniques:*** To improve taste and absorption, blend castor oil with other liquids or include it in your diet. Avoid exceeding suggested dosages to ensure a well-balanced incorporation into your daily routine.

5. ***Proper timing*** is crucial for maximizing castor oil's advantages. Some people like to take it in the morning on an empty stomach, while others find that it works best in the evening. Experiment to see what fits your body's rhythm.

6. *Listen to Your Body:* Observe how your body responds. Any unpleasant effects, such as nausea or pain, may suggest that the dosage should be adjusted or discontinued. Regular check-ins enable a smooth integration.

7. *Consult with experts:* Ask healthcare experts or nutritionists before using castor oil internally. They can provide you with tailored recommendations depending on your health situation and any potential contraindications.

Internal usage of castor oil can be both safe and useful with proper guidance. From choosing high-quality goods to monitoring your body's response, a cautious and knowledgeable approach assures a journey distinguished by wellness rather than unnecessary hazards.

Crafting Your Signature Castor Blends

.Making your own castor oil mixes gives you a plethora of options for tailored skincare and haircare regimens.

Understanding the many advantages of castor oil and mixing it with complimentary oils is essential for building a unique mixture.
Begin by using a high-quality, cold-pressed castor oil as the basis. This guarantees that you get the maximum benefit of its nutritious characteristics without compromising.

Castor oil is known for its moisturizing and conditioning properties, which promote healthy skin and hair.

Consider adding coconut oil for a subtle, tropical scent and increased moisture. Coconut oil enhances the richness of castor oil, resulting in a profoundly hydrating mix that does not feel heavy. It also gives your mix a velvety feel, making it a sensory joy.

To address specific skin conditions, use jojoba oil, which is recognized for its balancing characteristics. Jojoba oil resembles the skin's natural oils; therefore, it is excellent for all skin types.

This inclusion creates a balanced blend that leaves your skin feeling nourished and invigorated.

Almond oil can help increase hair growth. Almond oil, which is high in vitamins and minerals, helps to strengthen hair follicles in addition to castor oil. The end result is a powerful combination that promotes thicker, healthier hair.

Experiment with essential oils to personalize the smell and boost the therapeutic properties of your combination. Lavender oil has a relaxing effect, whilst peppermint oil stimulates the senses. Tailor the essential oil selection to your tastes and desired results.

Maintain a proper ratio in your mix to ensure that each component serves its purpose efficiently.

A basic recommendation is to use 70-80% castor oil as the foundation and the remaining amount for additional oils. This results in a well-rounded mix that optimizes the advantages of each element.

Making your personal castor blends is a voyage of self-discovery and care. Embrace castor oil's adaptability and experiment with different combinations until you find the ideal blend for your specific skincare and haircare requirements.

Chapter 5: Castor Oil's Influence on Mental Harmony

Castor oil, well-known for its numerous health advantages, has a positive impact on mental health as well. This natural elixir has been shown to significantly improve mental health and emotional equilibrium.

One important component of castor oil's effect on mental health is its high fatty acid content, notably ricinoleic acid. This chemical has anti-inflammatory characteristics that extend to the brain, which may reduce neuroinflammation.

A tranquil and inflammation-free brain promotes increased cognitive performance and emotional stability, providing an atmosphere of mental harmony.

Furthermore, the oil's hydrating effects extend to the scalp. A well-nourished scalp can improve hair health, perhaps relieving dandruff and itching. Relief from these bodily discomforts can help reduce stress, which in turn improves mental health.

In traditional medicine, castor oil has been associated with detoxification.

Small doses of castor oil are thought to cleanse the digestive tract, removing toxins that may contribute to brain fog and exhaustion.

A clearer mind frequently leads to increased attention and emotional resilience.Another way castor oil influences mental equilibrium is through its ceremonial use in massages.

The therapeutic act of massage may reduce tension, and when paired with the oil's nourishing characteristics, it provides a comprehensive method of relaxation.

This technique may provide a sense of tranquility and mental clarity.

Castor oil's impact on mental peace stems from its anti-inflammatory, cleansing, and nourishing characteristics.

Whether used physically or consumed, this natural medication has the ability to promote a balanced and serene state of mind, making it an important complement to holistic well-being practices.

Nurturing Mind-Body Synchrony

Nurturing mind-body synchrony is a comprehensive approach to well-being that stresses the interdependence of mental and physical health.

 In this effort, castor oil appears as a flexible ally, providing complete advantages that are consistent with this integrative worldview.

Stress reduction is an important aspect of mind-body synchronization, and castor oil can help with this. Its high fatty acid content, notably ricinoleic acid, has a relaxing impact on the neurological system, helping to relieve stress and improve mental balance.

This dual-action cure addresses both the mind and the body, promoting a healthy equilibrium.

Castor oil also has anti-inflammatory qualities, which help to maintain total bodily wellbeing. It helps to relieve physical discomfort and promotes a more relaxed mood by lowering inflammation.

This interaction between the physical and mental domains emphasizes the importance of mind-body synchronization, in which the relaxing effects on the body transfer into a calm state of mind.

Castor oil's effect on the mind-body link is enhanced when applied topically. Massaging this oil into the skin not only nourishes and moisturizes but also promotes mindfulness.

Self-massage creates a direct relationship between physical experience and cerebral calm, strengthening the interconnectedness of our well-being.

Mind-body synchronization is a never-ending journey in the world of holistic health, and castor oil is a reliable partner.

Castor oil embodies a distinct synergy that corresponds with the ideal of cultivating a harmonious connection between the mind and body, whether through its stress-relieving effects, anti-inflammatory benefits, or the contemplative act of self-massage.

Embracing this complete approach can lead to improved well-being and a more balanced, harmonious existence.

Castor Oil's Role in Stress Alleviation

Castor oil, which contains ricinoleic acid, has anti-inflammatory properties that help to reduce stress.

When administered topically or in massage, it increases blood circulation, promotes relaxation, and relieves muscle tension. Because of its dual impact on both the physical and mental levels, it is a comprehensive stress reliever.

Furthermore, castor oil is a nourishing ingredient for the skin. Its deep moisturizing properties not only promote better skin but also have a favorable effect on mood.

Hydrated skin corresponds with a sense of well-being, which has a knock-on impact that reduces stress levels.
The oil contains fatty acids, which play an important function in maintaining the neurological system. These important fatty

acids serve as neurotransmitter building blocks, helping to regulate mood and stress responses. Individuals who incorporate castor oil into their regimen may improve their emotional resilience and ability to cope with daily pressures.

In aromatherapy, castor oil's moderate smell can have a relaxing impact on the psyche.

Diffusing this oil in living spaces generates a relaxing atmosphere, providing a haven where tension may be relieved. The olfactory impact complements its topical treatments, resulting in a multisensory approach to stress alleviation.

Castor oil appears as a comprehensive stress-relieving agent. Its anti-inflammatory, hydrating, and neurotransmitter-supporting capabilities, as well as its aromatherapeutic advantages, all contribute to a holistic stress management plan.

Castor oil, whether used directly or diffused into the air, offers a natural and comprehensive approach to finding peace in the face of life's responsibilities.

Fostering Emotional Equilibrium

Fostering emotional stability is an important component of general well-being, and castor oil can help with this.

 While castor oil is well-known for its exterior applications, such as hair growth and skin health, it has also been connected to emotional equilibrium when consumed internally.

Castor oil, which contains the unusual fatty acid ricinoleic acid, is thought to impact serotonin receptors in the brain.

Serotonin, sometimes known as the "feel-good" neurotransmitter, regulates mood and emotions. Castor oil, by favorably interacting with serotonin receptors, may help to promote emotional stability.

Furthermore, castor oil contains omega-3 fatty acids, which might benefit brain function. These necessary fatty acids are recognized to provide cognitive advantages, including increased brain clarity and emotional resilience. A well-nourished brain can better handle stress and maintain emotional balance.

It's crucial to remember that, while castor oil may have some advantages, moderation is essential.

Excessive drinking might cause stomach pain and other negative consequences. Including tiny amounts of castor oil in a balanced diet may be a practical way to get its emotional well-being advantages.

The ritualistic self-care connected with castor oil use might help to maintain emotional equilibrium. Taking time for oneself and adopting holistic practices into everyday life can have a positive influence on mental health.

Fostering emotional stability requires a varied strategy, and castor oil, when used correctly, can be an unexpected ally.

Castor oil has the power to impact neurotransmitters and supply food to the brain, making it a unique tool for enhancing emotional well-being.

As with any wellness practice, it is recommended to contact a healthcare practitioner to confirm that it is appropriate for your specific requirements and circumstances.

Chapter 6: Unveiling Castor Oil's Expanded Horizons

Castor oil, a flexible and time-honored elixir, has lately announced new applications in a variety of sectors, demonstrating that it is more than simply a traditional treatment.

Beyond its well-known use, castor oil is making waves in the cosmetics, lubricants, and biofuel industries.

Castor oil has emerged as a popular cosmetic component among skincare lovers. Its natural moisturizing characteristics and high fatty acid content make it an excellent choice for hydrating skin and maintaining a healthy shine.

Castor oil-infused beauty products are well-known for their ability to restore hair, thicken lashes, and promote healthy eyebrows. As natural ingredients become more popular among customers, castor oil has evolved as a symbol of simplicity and efficacy in the cosmetics business.

Beyond the vanity mirror, castor oil has found application in the field of lubricants. Its viscosity and endurance make it an ideal choice for a variety of equipment applications.

Castor oil lubricants are proven to be dependable and ecological solutions for vehicle engines and industrial equipment. The inherent biodegradability of castor oil contributes to the global demand for ecologically friendly alternatives.

Furthermore, the renewable energy sector is seeing castor oil emerge as a crucial participant in biofuel production.

 As countries seek greener energy sources, castor oil's potential as a biodiesel feedstock has gained traction. Castor plants' propensity to grow in dry settings, along with their relative ease of cultivation, makes them a sustainable source of biofuel generation, helping to create a greener future.

Castor oil's expanding applications extend beyond its traditional functions, including cosmetics, lubricants, and biofuels.

As companies seek sustainable alternatives, castor oil stands out as a flexible option with a long history and a bright future.

Household Healing with Castor Oil

Castor oil, a versatile elixir with a long history, has emerged as a home healer, providing several advantages beyond its traditional usage. Its efficacy stems from its powerful characteristics, which promote healing and well-being.

1. *Skin savior:* Castor oil's moisturizing characteristics make it a skincare hero. Its deep moisturizing power combats dryness while minimizing the appearance of wrinkles and fine lines. When used topically, it calms inflamed skin and relieves a variety of dermatological issues.

2. *Hair Health Booster:* Castor oil is becoming a popular cure for restoring lustrous hair. As a natural conditioner, it promotes hair development, strengthens strands, and prevents split ends.

Regular scalp massages with castor oil promote healthier, shinier hair.

3. *Joint and Muscle Relief:* Castor oil's anti-inflammatory qualities help alleviate joint and muscle discomfort. Massaging the afflicted regions with heated castor oil improves circulation and relieves arthritis, painful muscles, and joint stiffness.

4. *Immune System Support:* Castor oil contains antioxidants that boost the immune system. Its antimicrobial capabilities combat infections, making it a dependable ally throughout seasonal changes or while feeling under the weather.

5. *Digestive Detox:* Castor oil has been used for ages as a natural treatment for digestive disorders. Consumed in moderation, it functions as a moderate laxative, encouraging bowel motions and assisting in detoxification.

6. *Castor oil's antibacterial properties* promote wound healing. When administered topically, it forms a protective barrier that prevents infections and promotes skin regeneration.

7. Enhance your natural attractiveness using castor oil for lashes and brows. Its nourishing characteristics promote thicker and longer development, making it a natural alternative for individuals who want lush lashes and well-defined brows.

Castor oil has grown into a household therapeutic treasure, providing a comprehensive approach to wellbeing.

From cosmetics to digestive health, its numerous uses make it an essential part of any home remedy repertoire.

Environmental Responsibility and Sustainability

Castor oil, a versatile and valuable resource, plays an important role in many sectors. However, the environmental effects of its manufacture necessitate a responsible approach to sustainability.

First and foremost, sustainable farming techniques are essential. Adopting organic agricultural practices reduces the need for synthetic pesticides and fertilizers, minimizing soil degradation and protecting biodiversity.

Precision agricultural approaches improve resource efficiency while minimizing water and energy consumption in castor oil growing.

Efficient extraction processes are critical to environmental responsibility. Using environmentally friendly extraction procedures, such as cold pressing, reduces energy consumption and chemical use.

This not only maintains the oil's quality but also considerably minimizes the carbon footprint connected with its production.

Waste management is another major issue. The responsible disposal or recycling of byproducts from castor oil production helps reduce environmental contamination.

Innovative solutions to recycle castor oil byproducts can help create a circular economy and promote sustainability across the supply chain.

In terms of packaging, using eco-friendly materials such as biodegradable or recyclable packaging demonstrates environmental commitment. This guarantees that the environmental impact of the product goes beyond production and throughout its full existence.

Furthermore, promoting fair trade practices promotes societal sustainability.

Fair salaries and ethical working conditions for castor oil producers help to improve the industry's overall environmental responsibility.

Attaining environmental responsibility and sustainability through castor oil manufacturing requires a comprehensive strategy.

Every component of the supply chain is important, from sustainable agricultural techniques to environmentally friendly extraction processes, waste management, and ethical labor standards.

Embracing these principles guarantees that castor oil remains a useful resource without jeopardizing our planet's health.

Narratives of Triumph with Castor Oil

Castor oil, a versatile elixir produced from the Ricinus communis plant, has emerged as a triumphant symbol in a variety of health and beauty storylines.

Its varied advantages have piqued the interest of those looking for natural solutions for a variety of issues.

In the world of hair care, castor oil is a symbol of victory over hair loss and dull strands. Its strong fatty acid content and nourishing characteristics help to strengthen hair follicles, promote hair growth, and prevent breakage.

Many people have praised castor oil's transforming potential in attaining thicker, healthier locks, marking a successful transition from hair difficulties to dazzling tresses.

Castor oil's tale also includes skin victories. This natural emollient works deep inside the skin, promoting moisture and combating dryness.

Countless people have observed castor oil's success in treating skin problems such as eczema and dermatitis, leaving behind a path of improved skin health.

Castor oil's emollient characteristics extend to skincare, where it has proven effective for people looking for a natural acne treatment. Its antibacterial properties battle microorganisms, and its fatty acids regulate oil synthesis.

Users have been amazed at the victory over acne outbreaks, enjoying smoother, healthier skin.

Beyond beauty, castor oil's success extends to overall wellness. Its well-known purgative properties have been used in ancient and traditional medicine to relieve constipation.

The victory over intestinal pain has established castor oil as a reliable therapy for sustaining general health.

The stories of success with castor oil are as varied as its applications. From hair and skin care to overall health, this natural wonder has carved out a place for itself in the quest for holistic well-being.

Its path from seed to solution is one of victory, welcomed by individuals seeking the astonishing advantages of a simple yet potent potion.

Chapter 7: Safeguarding Your Castor Journey

To ensure a smooth transition, begin introducing castor oil into your regimen with care. Consider the following crucial elements to ensure your caster voyage is safe:.

First and foremost, quality counts. Choose organic, cold-pressed castor oil to maintain purity and preserve its therapeutic characteristics.

This process of extraction protects the oil's nutrients while reducing the chance of contamination, resulting in a strong elixir for your hair, skin, and general health.

Next, moderation is essential. While castor oil has several advantages, it is important to use it in moderation. A weekly scalp massage with a diluted solution might promote hair growth without overpowering your strands. When it comes to skincare, a few drops blended with a carrier oil may do wonders without irritating the skin.

Timing is also important in optimizing the effects of castor oil. When applied before bedtime, the oil penetrates and nourishes your hair and skin overnight.

This overnight treatment harnesses castor oil's regenerative properties to promote healthier hair and a more luminous complexion.

Consistency is the key to success in your castor oil journey. Incorporate it into your daily regimen for long-term effects. Whether you want beautiful locks or bright skin, keeping to a consistent application regimen is essential to receiving the full benefits of castor oil.

Finally, have patience. Castor oil, like any other natural medicine, takes time to provide full results.

Allow your body and skin enough time to absorb and respond to castor oil's healing benefits. Patience mixed with consistency will produce the desired results.

Protecting your castor journey entails selecting high-quality products, applying them sparingly, scheduling applications carefully, keeping consistency, and practicing patience.

By following these suggestions, you may maximize the benefits of castor oil for a healthier, more vibrant you.

Unmasking Allergies and Sensitivities

Castor oil, despite its versatility and widespread usage, can nevertheless cause allergic responses and sensitivities in certain people.

Unraveling the complexities of these reactions is critical for a thorough knowledge of castor oil's effects on health.

Castor oil allergies are rare, but they can appear in a variety of ways. Skin responses, including redness, itching, and hives, are frequent symptoms.

Some people may have respiratory difficulties, such as trouble breathing or a runny nose, indicating the possibility of inhalation allergies.

It is critical to understand that allergic responses to castor oil can range in intensity from minor discomfort to severe anaphylaxis, which requires rapid medical assistance.

Castor oil sensitivities are less severe than allergies, yet they can still cause problems. Individuals with sensitive skin may experience discomfort or inflammation when in contact with castor oil-containing products.

Furthermore, gastrointestinal sensitivities might cause stomach pain or diarrhea when castor oil is used.

Identifying the source of castor oil might also help us understand allergic or sensitive reactions. While the oil itself is the main issue, any additives or impurities injected during production might worsen negative reactions.
Choosing high-quality, pure castor oil products and carefully reading ingredient labels helps reduce the chance of adverse effects.

Individuals must take proactive steps to identify and manage any castor oil allergies or sensitivities.

Patch testing can help determine skin reactions, but monitoring stomach and respiratory responses following exposure is critical.

Those with known allergies or sensitivities should consult with a healthcare practitioner before using castor oil-containing products.

While castor oil has various advantages, it is critical to recognize and manage the risk of allergies and sensitivities.

A sophisticated understanding of individual sensitivities, along with informed product selections, enables people to get the benefits of castor oil without jeopardizing their health.

*Safe Paths for Little Ones and
Expectant Mothers*

When evaluating the use of castor oil, it is critical to prioritize the safety of infants and pregnant women. Although it is a versatile drug, caution and attentiveness are required.

The use of castor oil to induce labor is a contentious issue among expecting moms. Some swear by its effectiveness, while others are concerned about its potential adverse effects.

When it comes to children, keep castor oil out of their reach. Its laxative qualities might be dangerous if used mistakenly. Childproof storage and attentive supervision are essential safeguards.

Furthermore, investigate alternatives for popular applications. Instead of exposing sensitive skin to the strength of castor oil, use softer oils for massages or moisturizing.

Expectant moms should approach the use of castor oil to induce labor with caution. While some anecdotal data shows that it might cause contractions, medical experts frequently advise against use owing to the possible hazards.

It is critical to contact a healthcare expert before using this procedure, since they may give individualized advice depending on specific health issues.

Dilution is essential in skin care regimes for both young children and expecting women. Mix castor oil with a carrier oil to make it mild on the skin.

Pregnant women, in particular, should exercise caution while using castor oil-based skincare products and instead choose formulas tailored to their specific needs.

While castor oil offers benefits, it is important to use caution, especially when dealing with children and pregnant women. Prioritize safety by keeping it out of reach, researching alternative products, and communicating with healthcare specialists for specific recommendations.

Dilution and moderation are the keys to realizing castor oil's potential advantages while protecting the well-being of our community's most vulnerable individuals.

The Collaborative Approach – Consulting Healthcare Professionals

Collaboration between healthcare providers and patients is essential for making educated decisions about using castor oil.

This natural treatment, made from the seeds of the Ricinus communis plant, has received attention due to its possible health advantages. However, a coordinated approach is required to guarantee safe and effective use.

Healthcare professionals play an important role in educating patients about the correct use of castor oil. They have the knowledge to evaluate individual health situations, potential contraindications, and dose requirements.

Professionals who communicate openly with patients may address their issues and make individualized recommendations, improving the entire therapy experience.

Healthcare practitioners should promote castor oil's historic usage as well as current study findings. While it has traditionally been used for its laxative characteristics, current research suggests that it may also have anti-inflammatory and skin-nourishing benefits.

This collaborative conversation empowers patients to make educated decisions based on a comprehensive understanding of the advantages of castor oil.

Furthermore, healthcare providers should educate patients about the significance of quality assurance when choosing castor oil products. Variations in processing processes and purity levels can have an influence on efficacy and safety. Individuals may navigate product selections by talking with healthcare specialists, ensuring they choose reputed products that meet quality requirements.

When it comes to the use of castor oil, healthcare professionals and patients must work together. This offers a thorough grasp of its possible advantages, tailored suggestions based on specific health variables, and assistance in selecting high-quality items.

By encouraging open communication, healthcare providers enable patients to make educated decisions, enabling the safe and successful incorporation of castor oil into their wellness routines.

CONCLUSION

In this book, a tapestry of enlightenment develops, weaving together the historical knowledge and modern significance of castor oil.

At its core, this comprehensive book goes beyond the norm, welcoming newcomers into a realm where healing wisdom meets practical health applications.

The voyage begins with a historical excursion to discover the origins of castor oil and its tremendous significance in diverse civilizations.

This contextual grounding not only provides depth but also emphasizes castor oil's time-tested therapeutic properties. From ancient cures to current medicinal techniques, the guide elegantly bridges the chronological divide, cultivating an appreciation for castor oil's long-lasting usefulness.

The guide's genius stems from its ability to simplify complicated knowledge into understandable concepts, making it a helpful resource for newbies.

Readers are exposed to the various applications of castor oil, from beauty regimens to digestive assistance, as well as its ability to promote hair health, through concise explanations.

The book acts as a road map for newbies, helping them to confidently explore the vast landscape of castor oil advantages.

Practicality is key in this book, and the inclusion of beginner-friendly recommendations ensures that readers can easily include castor oil into their daily wellness routines. Whether it's demystifying the technique of oil pulling or offering step-by-step directions for making nourishing hair masks, the guide enables people to utilize the entire range of castor oil's restorative properties.

"This book" is more than just an instructional guide; it's an empowering companion for everyone beginning on a path of holistic well-being.

By combining old knowledge with modern insights, the book becomes a lighthouse, illuminating the road to balanced life and rejuvenation.

In short, the book contains not only the wonders of castor oil, but also the transforming power it possesses for anyone wishing to integrate healing wisdom into their everyday lives.

THANK YOU PAGE

Thank you for selecting the castor oil Wonders, a versatile and healthy product. Your support is really appreciated. Similarly, I am grateful for the purchase of this book.

Your input is valuable; please share your ideas in a review. It serves as a reference for future improvements. Enjoy reading and utilizing it!